What Men Won't Talk About
...and Women Need to Know

With hope & hugs

[signature]

What Men Won't Talk About
...and Women Need to Know

A Woman's Perspective on Prostate Cancer

Glenda Standeven

www.IamChoosingToSmile.com

Standeven Publications
9872 Candow Street
Chilliwack, BC
V2P 4K4
Canada

www.IAmChoosingToSmile.com
www.glendastandeven.com

Printed in Canada

ISBN: 978-0-9813307-1-6

FIRST EDITION
17 16 15 14   10 9 8 7 6 5 4 3 2 1

The information in this book is not meant to replace the care given by an expert medical practitioner but we hope it will be used as a tool to aid prostate cancer patients and their spouses in their quest for information.

Designer: Detta Penna
Proofreader: Wendy Dewar-Hughes; Summer Bay Press
Cover photo and author photos: Courtesy of Taichi Maehata

This book is dedicated to my wonderful husband, Rick,
and to all the brave men who face
prostate cancer,
and especially to my dad, Barney Bobroske,
who taught us so much through his own journey.

Contents

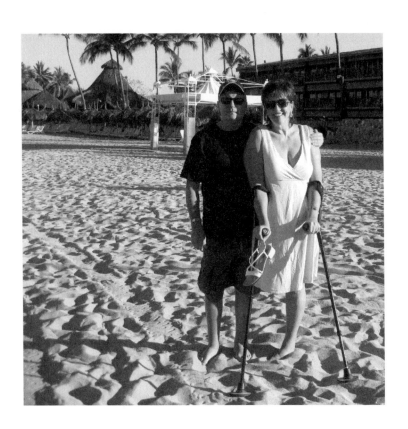

Foreword

I am, among other things, wife, mother, cancer survivor, amputee, author, and inspirational speaker. In 2009, I co-authored a book called *Choosing to Smile*. It was written with two close friends who, like me, had also been diagnosed with cancer. We hoped that by sharing our stories we would help others to face their own challenges with a positive attitude. After writing and successfully publishing our book, I never dreamed that my wonderful husband would all too soon be facing his own adversity that would test the foundations of our choosing to smile philosophy.

What Men Won't Talk About and Women Need to Know was written out of necessity. My husband and I have been married since 1982, and, over the years, he has shown me that there are many things a man is eager and willing to do to please a woman, but going for a prostate exam isn't one of them! It is my sincere hope that this little book will enlighten both men and women and, in the process, perhaps save lives by shedding some light on a topic that many men feel is taboo. This book is also for women everywhere—because sometimes our men need to be reminded about what our wants and needs are too. First and foremost, we want and need the special men in our lives to LIVE.

Chapter One

The Warning Signs

"Come on, Rick! You've got to be able to pee harder than that!" I was lying in bed with my head cocked to one side, listening intently to the sounds coming from the adjoining bathroom. My husband valiantly attempted to satisfy my apparent need to hear him pee long and loud—like a fire hose turned loose in the bowl. It wasn't working. His stream sounded more like an annoying faucet leaking and dribbling than the thundering pee waterfall I wanted to hear. I wanted to hear the kind of pee that left bubbles bouncing in the bowl.

I had noticed, with a sense of increasing worry, that he seemed to hesitate and concentrated harder on the task when he stood in front of a toilet. I, on the other hand, just had to come within eyesight of a toilet and I'd start to pee—whether I wanted to or not! Oh, the joys of growing older. But something was bothering me about my husband's condition and a little voice kept telling me that something was seriously wrong. I've learned to listen to that voice.

My father was diagnosed on Valentine's Day, 1992, and he passed away from metastatic prostate cancer in March, 1993. I learned a lot from his journey, and I give him credit for making me aware of the warning signs. He was only 65 years old when he was diagnosed with terminal prostate cancer. It had already metastasized by the time they discovered it. Or should I say, by the time he decided to do something about it.

I have discovered that a lot of men don't like to discuss their serious illnesses. Many men take it as a sign of weakness to be ill, but I was determined that my husband would never fall into that category. I would hustle him into the doctor's office at the first hint that something wasn't right. It's not that I'm a hypochondriac, because I'm not. Neurotic maybe. But I have reason to be. I lost my entire right leg, including my hip and pelvis, to a very aggressive bone cancer (chondrosarcoma) in 1988, when I was 32 years old. The doctors originally thought it was bursitis so now I tend to pay attention when my body doesn't feel right. And I guess that watchfulness has spilled over to those closest to me.

For example, paying attention saved my husband's life in 2006, when I discovered a malignant melanoma skin cancer growing on his left forearm. His "trucker" arm was deeply tanned and, as I was idly running my fingers up and down his arm one night, I noticed a rough, two-toned mole that I'd never felt before. Sure enough, the innocuous little spot that he was sure was "nothing" turned out to be melanoma—a potentially deadly skin cancer. Fortunately, we caught it at the earliest stage possible—in situ—which means the tumour cells are still confined to the site where they originated and they have neither invaded neighbouring tissues nor metastasized. My own cancer journey taught me all sorts of useful health tips like knowing the difference between a mole that is harmless and one that potentially isn't. My father's cancer journey taught me what warning signs* to watch for when it came to my husband's prostate health concerns.

*See *Things You Need To Know and Helpful Tips* for a detailed list of warning signs.

"Honey, I don't know what you expect. I'm not a kid anymore. I can't pee like I did when I was 17 you know." Each sentence my husband spoke was an exclamation of not only his frustration with not being able to muster up a good head in the bowl anymore but also his frustration with having an audience listening when he *did* have to pee.

"I'm sorry for nagging, Rick, but I'm worried. And how many times did you get up last night to pee?" Much to Rick's dismay, I was like a dog with a bone and wouldn't let it go.

I heard his heavy sigh coming from the bathroom, "Five or six maybe. Who's counting?"

"Apparently I am! I'm making an appointment for you. You're due for another PSA (Prostate Specific Antigen) test anyway."

And so it began.

Chapter Two

The Diagnosis

Rick went for his annual blood work, and in October we sat in the doctor's office as she went over his PSA results with us. Rick had been having annual digital rectal exams (DRE) and PSA blood tests done since my dad's death as an extra precautionary measure. We had to pay for the PSA tests at that time because he was considered too young to be at any serious risk of the disease but it was $40 well spent, as far as I was concerned. At some point in his fifties our family doctor decided to order Rick's PSA, and the tests were covered under our medical plan but, even if they hadn't been covered, we would still have paid gladly for this lifesaving test.

"So, I'm a little concerned with the results of the PSA test this time." We weren't really expecting to hear those words coming from our doctor's mouth and I felt my breath catch in my throat. "Normal PSA is 4.0 or less and yours is 1.8." Whew. I felt myself begin to exhale with relief but caught it again when she paused. Rick was well within the normal range so why did I suddenly feel anxious? I felt a tightness in my chest and I knew that the pause was going to be followed by one of my least favourite words— "but." I was right.

"But your count has doubled since the last test a year ago and it should never double even if it's still low. You went from 0.8 to 1.6 and I'd like you to see a urologist just to make sure everything is okay." I blessed her for being on top of her game because I have a hunch not every doctor would have caught that little jump in his numbers.

There's a lesson here, men—it's so important to know what your PSA numbers are. It's not enough just to have the test done and leave it up to your physician to monitor the results. You need to *know* what the numbers mean and *know* what is normal and abnormal. Some studies are suggesting that PSA tests are not necessary or that they are inconclusive, but I know for a fact that having an annual PSA test gave us a baseline to go on and that one simple thing could now possibly save my husband's life.

Our doctor made the appointment to see the urologist and the fact that we got in to see him in less than a month had me a little concerned. In my experience, when things in the medical world move quickly it's never a good sign! On Friday, November 25, we went to see the specialist. He looked at Rick's numbers and asked with unveiled surprise why we were even there. He explained that with numbers that low there was only a thirty-five percent chance or less of it being prostate cancer. He sort of shrugged and said, "But I can do a biopsy if it will make you feel better."

I looked at the doctor in disbelief. "Heck, *yes!* If someone gave me a thirty-five percent chance of winning the lottery I guarantee you I'd buy a ticket." Poor Rick. I think the protective wife instinct in me came out ready to fight before he could even process what the doctor was saying. When you suspect it could be something serious you should always have a second person with you whenever you see a doctor. From past experience of dealing with my own cancer diagnosis, I remember that I could see their mouths moving but I stopped hearing the moment I heard the word "cancer" so I always appreciated having a second set of ears at my appointments to catch what I missed. That's why I never let Rick go to a doctor appointment alone. Neurotic? Maybe—but I'm not a hypochondriac.

You also need to be aware that before they do the biopsy, your rectum needs to be as clean as a whistle to prevent the possibility of infection. You won't be straying far from home after drinking the bowel preparation the day before surgery, but I don't think a good cleanout ever hurt anyone. Rick took antibiotic pills starting a day before the biopsy and for the following week, just as an added measure to ward off any chance of infection after having the procedure.

Rick had a ten-needle biopsy at the Chilliwack General Hospital on December 19th, 2011. He says it was most definitely *not* a pleasant experience but not the worst either. He described it as both a stinging sensation and a burn at the same time. They can't really freeze the prostate, and to get to it they have to go through the rectum and insert a needle through the bowel wall into the prostate gland to take a sample for biopsy purposes. He was awake for the procedure but wished he had been knocked out by the time the tenth sample was taken. But the worst thing was that the doctor said Rick couldn't have sex or any kind of "release" for a week after the procedure. Rick and I enjoyed an active sex life so he wasn't too happy with that news. I assured him we'd survive.

We have had men talk to us after hearing that Rick had prostate cancer and tell us that they know they are okay because they've had a colonoscopy done.

No, you are not necessarily okay!

A colonoscopy and a prostate exam are two completely different things. If you look on the diagram on the next page, you will see where the prostate is located.

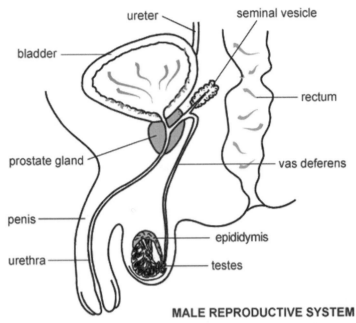

ureter

seminal vesicle

bladder

rectum

prostate gland

vas deferens

penis

epididymis

urethra

testes

MALE REPRODUCTIVE SYSTEM

A colonoscopy looks for signs of colon cancer, and a DRE (Digital Rectal Exam) looks for changes in your prostate by inserting a gloved finger into the rectum and feeling the surface of the prostate through the rectum wall. I imagine it would be like putting a thick piece of plastic over a walnut and trying to visualize if it's a normal-shaped nut or not. If the prostate is enlarged, lumpy, hard, or misshapen, a DRE will let the physician know that something is potentially amiss and the doctor will book more tests to confirm a diagnosis.

The biopsy procedure didn't take long but the aftereffects were surprising. Over the next few days, when he peed, Rick's urine was tinged with blood and small blood clots came out with it. We did wait the required week before having sex and, with some trepidation, we noticed that the semen was bloody, which was not very erotic or sexy for either of us. The blood-tinged ejaculate probably lasted a good three weeks but we simply used a condom until the problem resolved. Where there's a will there is generally—but not always—a way. Rick didn't even miss a day of work after the biopsy. What a trooper!

Christmas was just around the corner. I think we were both having flashbacks to my own cancer biopsy results which had arrived on December 22, 1987. When our family doctor phoned and asked us to come in (on her day off) to talk to us about Rick's biopsy results we both refused to believe a cancer diagnosis could happen. It was Friday, December 23, 2011, and we *almost* had ourselves convinced that there was no way we could be getting bad news this close to Christmas because, well, that would just suck.

But of course, if you've had any life experience at all, you know that sometimes things just don't pan out the way you hope, plan, or expect them to. This was no exception. My husband took the news better than I did when our doctor sombrely said, "I'm sort of shocked but the biopsy was positive for cancer. I really didn't think it would be cancer, but two of the ten samples came back positive. There's a scale they use to determine the seriousness of the cancer. It's called a Gleason Scale* and it rates prostate cancer on a scale from 1 to 10; 5 being low level and 10 being the most severe. Your scores came back as a 6 and a 7."

Well, that just sucks, doesn't it.

---

*details about how a Gleason score is achieved are found in *Things You Need To Know and Helpful Tips* at the back of the book.

Chapter Three

The Options

Rick and I were both stunned. We had really been hoping for the best, and here we were getting the worst. Ever the optimist, I grasped at straws and said, "Well, it could be worse—it could be a level 9 and 10 and it's not." That was small comfort but neither of us are quitters, so we held on to anything positive we could find in the situation.

"So now what do we do?" my husband asked. We both wanted and needed an action plan.

"Well, I'll make an appointment for you at the Cancer Centre in Abbotsford with a radiologist who will go over some of your treatment options. You should see the surgeon again as well to discuss surgery options."

Hmm, both were very practical next steps but all I was hearing was, "blah blah blah CANCER blah blah blah" and I was supposed to be the one taking notes.

"You're booked to see the surgeon next week to go over the biopsy results but I'll get the other appointment for you as soon as possible." She obviously understood that waiting for treatment was the worst part after the initial diagnosis.

Mustering what inner strength I could, I squeezed Rick's hand and said, "Let's not tell our families until after Christmas. There's no point in ruining Christmas for everyone." Rick nodded. He was obviously still processing the information we'd just been given. He told me later that all he could think about was how my dad and his step-dad, Moe, had both passed away from the same disease he'd just been told that he had. I can only imagine how frightened he must have felt inside and how brave he appeared on the outside. At least until we got into the car.

We sat in the car—too stunned to drive home yet. We hugged each other hard across the console and I couldn't stop the tears. Rick's eyes grew moist as he held me in his arms and reassured me that he had no intention of dying just yet. "We have a lot of living to do honey. We caught it early. I don't look or feel sick. We'll get through this!" I repeated the words of comfort that rushed from his mouth.

"You're young and strong. If anyone can beat cancer, it's you! We'll do this together, honey!" We knew we were both spewing platitudes but we weren't ready to get down and dirty with the reality of the disease yet. After all, Christmas was just two days away.

Christmas passed in a whirlwind of emotions for both of us. We tried to hold on to each precious second of happiness as every smile became more special and every laugh became more treasured. That is one of the gifts that cancer gave us that Christmas— an added appreciation for everyday joys. Our families and friends were oblivious to the worry Rick and I carried inside. We were too busy making memories to let cancer steal even a minute of anyone else's Christmas spirit. Our resolve to fight was strengthened by both of our wonderful families over the holidays.

Thursday, December 29, 2011, we sat in the urologist's office going over Rick's surgical options. We didn't like what we were hearing. "With a PSA of 1.6 I never would have suspected the growth would be a level 6 and 7 on the Gleason Scale. I'm just as surprised as you are. Fortunately, the two positive biopsy samples came from the same quadrant so it doesn't appear to have spread to the entire prostate. I recommend a radical prostatectomy, where we surgically remove the entire prostate."

I interrupted him by asking the question that had been on both Rick's and my mind since we found out he had prostate cancer. "Um, what about his ability to have an erection after the surgery? We've heard about a procedure that can remove the prostate but still spare the nerves."

"Yes, there is such a thing as a nerve-sparing radical prostatectomy *(See the note at the end of this chapter),* but he likely won't be able to have an erection. We can discuss that later."

We didn't want to discuss it later. We wanted to discuss it now, and we also decided we wanted a second opinion. Please note that you are *entitled* to a second opinion so, if you're not 100% comfortable with your medical support team, don't be afraid or hesitant to ask to see someone else. You can always go back once you've weighed your options and made an educated decision.

We knew there was a Vancouver Prostate Centre just an hour from home, where their sole purpose was looking after men's prostate health so we decided to make an appointment there. We felt time was on our side because his PSA was, indeed, so low. We were wrong, of course, to rely on that little number.

The Web becomes your best friend and also your worst enemy when you have a serious illness. We learned to find legitimate websites and avoided the ones that wanted to sell us something. We learned more than we ever wanted to know about prostate cancer. We also sought reviews for doctors and surgeons at the Vancouver Prostate Centre and decided we wanted to see Dr. Alan So for a second opinion. We booked an appointment for February 1, 2012, and we were excited to meet the man who had so many great patient reviews, but we dreaded the job of telling our family that we would be facing another cancer hurdle in the new year.

We needn't have worried. Our two sons were pillars of strength, and our families and friends all handled the news with calm reassurances that they would support us through our journey in any way they could. If they doubted that Rick would beat cancer they certainly never let us see their fears. I bless them for their strength because it helped us get through the upcoming challenges a lot easier without expending any precious energy worrying about them and how they were coping with his illness.

It took a little over a month to get an appointment to see the radiation oncologist at the Cancer Centre in Abbotsford. He was honest, patient, and gave us more than enough information to make an educated decision about which option we should choose. He explained the benefits and risks of both external radiation and Brachytherapy where small radioactive pellets are inserted into the prostate gland. The way we understood it, in external radiation the radiation had to travel through healthy tissue to get to the bad. The prostate cancer is destroyed by the radiation but so is healthy tissue. In both Brachytherapy and external radiation treatments the prostate would eventually become non-functioning and harden. And, if the radiation extended beyond the prostate, healthy tissue would be damaged, which would make nerve-sparing surgery at a later date no longer an option. Radiation could also cause bowel problems because the prostate is in such close proximity to the bowel area. Neither option appealed to us and, thankfully, because of Rick's age and the surprisingly high Gleason score, the radiation oncologist agreed that radiation might not be our best option. Some men are also able to consider hormone therapy to slow the tumour growth, but Rick wasn't a good candidate for that either because of his young age and the aggressive nature of his tumour. That made surgery our only other choice.

On February 1, 2012, we met with Dr. So at the Vancouver Prostate Centre. As soon as we sat down in the chairs across from his desk he said, "Well, I bet you're wondering about erections!" Of course we liked him immediately. He was young, handsome, confident, and patient. He took time to show us diagrams to explain the prostatectomy procedure. He handed us a bundle of pamphlets to read and told Rick to be sure and practice his Kegel* exercises both before and after his surgery. Rick didn't really know what a Kegel was so *(big mistake)* he never spent any time or effort to learn how to do a Kegel exercise properly. This little omission would come back to bite him on the butt after the surgery!

Dr. So assured us that he would do his very best to spare the two delicate bundles of nerves that run alongside the prostate gland. These two innocuous little nerve bundles control the ability to have an erection and that was an ability Rick wasn't quite ready to relinquish to cancer. Dr. So suggested we take a nice vacation before the surgery and spend some quality time together (I think that was his code for making love like crazy). He booked the surgery for May 1. Rick would finish his job working on the winter road maintenance crew on March 15, 2012, and my work commitments were done at the end of March, so we booked an adventure vacation in Puerto Vallarta, Mexico, for the first two weeks

---

*Read detailed instructions for Kegel exercises in *Things You Need To Know and Helpful Tips* at the back of the book.

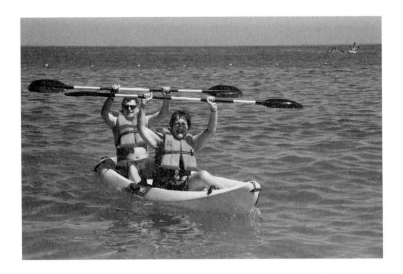

of April. It was going to be an amazing month filled with making memories and making love. We kept a little blessings book where we wrote down all the special things that happened during our vacation. The pages filled rapidly. We truly felt that our vacation was blessed from start to finish and I highly recommend that you keep a blessings book handy throughout your prostate cancer journey. It helps so much to focus on the positive things that happen rather than the negative.

In Mexico, we swam with dolphins and sea lions, snorkelled, boogie-boarded, kayaked on the ocean, held a monkey, kissed a parrot, parasailed, rode on a catamaran, took a riverboat ride to look for crocodiles, drank tequila, had couples massages under tents on the beach, and made love almost every day. It was absolutely the best vacation we could ever have imagined.

When we came home we had a few days to wash clothes and repack our suitcases to head to the Cancer Awareness Conference in Saskatoon, Saskatchewan, where I was a keynote speaker. One

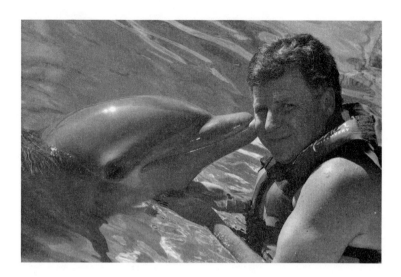

of the workshops we attended was led by an amazing Nurse Practitioner,* Reanne Booker, whose focus was on sexuality and cancer. She taught us more about what to expect after the surgery than any of our online sources. I bless her for being there and for being so open and honest about sex being natural, healthy, and important for *both* partners. By the time we got home from the conference we were optimistic and prepared, we thought, for the upcoming surgery and all that it would entail.

Funny how things can go sideways no matter how optimistic and prepared you think you are.

---

*A Nurse Practitioner (NP) is an advanced practice nurse who has completed additional education and training and has an expanded scope of practice. NPs can order diagnostic tests (labs, imaging, etc.), diagnose, prescribe interventions (including medications).

Note

A radical prostatectomy is an operation to remove the prostate gland and some of the tissue around it. It is done to remove prostate cancer. This operation may be done by open surgery. Or it may be done by laparoscopic surgery through small incisions.

Laparoscopic surgery may be done by hand. But some doctors now do it by guiding robotic arms that hold the surgery tools. This is called robot-assisted prostatectomy.

Open surgery

In open surgery, the surgeon makes an incision to reach the prostate gland. Depending on the case, the incision is made either in the lower belly or in the perineum between the anus and the scrotum.

When the incision is made in the lower belly, it is called the retro-pubic approach. In this procedure, the surgeon may also remove lymph nodes in the area so that they can be tested for cancer.

When the incision is made in the perineum, it is called the perineal approach. The recovery time after this surgery may be shorter than with the retro-pubic approach. If the surgeon wants to remove lymph nodes for testing, he or she must make a separate incision. If the lymph nodes are believed to be free of cancer based on the grade of the cancer and results of the PSA test, the surgeon may not remove lymph nodes.

Laparoscopic surgery

For laparoscopic surgery, the surgeon makes several small incisions in the belly. A lighted viewing instrument called a laparoscope is inserted into one of the incisions. The surgeon uses special instruments to reach and remove the prostate through the other incisions.

Robotic-assisted laparoscopic radical prostatectomy is surgery done through small incisions in the belly with robotic arms that translate the surgeon's hand motions into finer and more precise action. This surgery requires specially-trained doctors.

The main goal of either open or laparoscopic surgery is to remove all the cancer. Sometimes that means removing the prostate and the tissues around it, including a set of nerves to the penis that affect the man's ability to have an erection. Some tumours can be removed using a nerve-sparing technique. This means carefully cutting around those nerves to leave them intact. Nerve-sparing surgery sometimes preserves the man's ability to have an erection.

What To Expect After Surgery

Prostatectomy usually requires general anaesthesia and a hospital stay of two to four days. A thin, flexible tube called a catheter usually is left in the bladder to drain urine for one to three weeks. Your doctor will give you instructions about how to care for your catheter at home. Bladder control can be poor for a few months after the catheter is removed.

Although prostatectomy often removes all cancer cells, be sure to get follow-up care, which may lead to early detection and treatment if your cancer comes back. Your regular follow-up program may include:

Physical exams

- Prostate-specific antigen (PSA) tests, to watch PSA levels and to measure the speed of any changes in those levels
- Digital rectal exams
- Biopsies, as needed, to look at suspicious tissue

Why It Is Done

Radical prostatectomy is most often used if testing shows that the cancer has not spread outside the prostate (Stages I and II). Radical prostatectomy is sometimes used to relieve urinary obstruction in men with more advanced (Stage III) cancer. But a different operation, called a transurethral resection of the prostate (TURP), is most often used for that purpose. Surgery is not usually considered a cure for advanced cancer, but it can help relieve symptoms.

How Well It Works

Radical prostatectomy is generally effective in treating prostate cancer that has not spread. This is called early-stage cancer. Following surgery, the stage of the cancer can be determined based on how far it has spread. PSA levels will drop almost to zero if the surgery successfully removes the cancer and the cancer has not spread. If cancer has spread, advanced cancer may develop even after the prostate has been removed.

For men younger than 65 with early stage cancer (Stages I and II, also called localized prostate cancer), those who had surgery lived longer than those who used active surveillance. For men older than 65 with early stage cancer, those who chose surgery lived just as long as men who chose other treatments, including active surveillance.

Studies show that how well you come through the surgery and the extent of your side effects depend more on the skill of your surgeon than on the kind of surgery you have.

Risks

Erection problems

Erection problems are one of the serious side effects of radical prostatectomy. The nerves that control a man's ability to have an erection lie next to the prostate gland. They often are damaged or removed during surgery. Sometimes these nerves can be spared during surgery to preserve erections.

About half of men are able to regain some of their ability to have erections, but this takes time. It can take as little as three months. But for most men, it will be six months to a year.

Recovery depends on: whether the man was able to have an erection before surgery; how the surgery affected the nerves that control erections; and how old the man was at the time of surgery

Medicines such as sildenafil (Viagra®), vardenafil (Levitra®), or tadalafil (Cialis®) and mechanical aids such as a penile pump may help men who are impotent because of treatment. Using medicines soon after surgery may help men regain sexual function. Talk with your doctor about your situation.

Urinary incontinence

Up to half of all men who have a radical prostatectomy develop urinary incontinence, ranging from a need to wear urinary incontinence pads to occasional dribbling. Studies show that one year later, between 15% and 50% of men report urinary problems.

The urethra, the tube that carries urine from your bladder, runs through the middle of the doughnut-shaped prostate gland. In order to remove the prostate, the surgeon must cut the urethra and later reconnect it to the bladder. Evidence shows that the greater the surgeon's experience and skill in making this reconnection, the lower the rate of incontinence.

Some men may need treatment for incontinence after prostatectomy, if urinary leakage continues longer than a year.

Complications

Radical prostatectomy is major surgery. It carries the same general risks as other major operations, including heart problems, blood clots, allergic reaction to anaesthesia, blood loss, and infection of the wound.

Also, these complications can be caused by radical prostatectomy: erection problems; urinary incontinence; damage to the urethra; damage to the rectum.

What To Think About

When considering prostatectomy, take into account your personal wishes, age, other medical conditions you may have, the stage and grade of your cancer, and your PSA level. Your age and overall health will make a difference in how treatment may affect your quality of life. Any health problems you have before treatment, especially urinary, bowel, or sexual function problems, will affect your recovery. Depending on your situation, active surveillance or radiation therapy may be reasonable options.

If you and your doctor decide that you need surgery, be sure to choose a highly skilled surgeon at a hospital that has a good success rate. Studies show that men have fewer side effects from prostate surgery when they have a skilled and experienced surgeon.

Robot-assisted prostatectomy may be best suited to a younger man in good health who has a small prostate and a small, lower-grade cancer.

Both surgery and radiation can cause urinary incontinence (not being able to control urination) or impotence (not being able to have an erection). The level of urinary incontinence and how long it lasts and the quality of the erections a man has after treatment will depend on whether the cancer has spread. These also depend on what treatment is used.

Surgery may completely remove your prostate cancer. It is not possible to know ahead of time whether the cancer has spread beyond the prostate and is not curable with surgery alone.

Citations

Lu-Yao, G. L., et al. (2010). Outcomes of localized prostate cancer following conservative management. JAMA, 302(11): 1202-1209.

Zelefsky, M. J., et al. (2008). Cancer of the prostate. In VT DeVita Jr et al., eds., Devita, Hellman, and Rosenberg's Cancer: Principles and Practice of Oncology, 8th ed., vol. 1, pp. 1392-1452. Philadelphia: Lippincott Williams and Wilkins.

National Cancer Institute (2010). Prostate Cancer Treatment (PDQ)-Health Professional Version. Available online: http://www.nci.nih.gov/cancertopics/pdq/treatment/prostate/healthprofessional.

Walsh, P. C., Partin, A. W. (2007). Anatomic radical retropubic prostatectomy. In A. J. Wein et al., eds., Campbell-Walsh *Urology*, 9th ed., vol. 3, pp. 2956-2978. Philadelphia: Saunders Elsevier.

James, M. L. (2006). Prostate cancer (early), search date February 2006. Online version of BMJ Clinical Evidence: http://www.clinicalevidence.com.

Kantoff, P. W. (2007). Prostate cancer. In D. C. Dale, D. D. Federman, eds., ACP Medicine, section 12, chap. 9. New York: WebMD.

Agency for Healthcare Research and Quality (2008). Comparative Effectiveness of Therapies for Clinically Localized Prostate Cancer: Executive Summary (AHRQ Pub. No. 08-EHC010-1). Rockville, MD: Agency for Healthcare Research and Quality. Available online: http://www.effectivehealthcare.ahrq.gov/ehc/products/9/79/2008_0204prostatecancerexecsum.pdf.

Chapter Four

The Surgery

We checked into a hotel next to St. Paul's Hospital in downtown Vancouver the night before the surgery, and made love one last time. I choked back tears because I knew what it meant for Rick to give up, as he was fond of saying, "Honey, [this is] the one thing I'm really good at!" He clung to the hope that the cancer had not spread beyond the prostate and that the nerve-sparing surgery would be a success, but I was just hoping he'd live. We spent a mostly sleepless night wrapped in each others' arms, dreading the morning.

We checked in early and went through all the motions of pre-admission for his upcoming surgery. Rick changed into the hospital gown and we sat waiting with a room full of quiet strangers all facing their own battles. We held hands and whispered confident words of support to each other. In an attempt to lighten our moods, I pulled a pen from my purse and said, "Hey, how about if I write on your stomach SPARE THE NERVES just to remind Dr. So of what we want?" Rick laughed but before we could do it, Dr. So joined us in the waiting room.

"Well, are you ready for the surgery?" He seemed so young and confident. Rick was placing his life in this man's hands, but no surgery should be taken lightly—especially one involving a man's private parts!

"My wife was just about to write a message on my stomach for you to read during surgery." Rick told him what I had wanted to do with the pen.

Dr. So smiled at me then turned to Rick and looked him directly in the eyes as he said slowly and clearly, "Cancer first. Nerves second." It was reassuring to know he had his priorities straight, even if ours were a little askew.

With a big hug and a kiss from me, Rick was led into the surgery ward. He seemed resigned and showed no signs of the worry I was feeling. I had thought it would be three or four hours, but five hours later I was still waiting to hear how the surgery went.

Finally Dr. So came out and told me, "The surgery went well and from what I could see the cancer has not moved beyond the prostate. The pathology report will confirm my findings. I took out the seminal vesicles and some lymph nodes to test as well. You'll be happy to know I was able to spare the nerves," he paused and I knew there was a big *"but"* about to drop out of his mouth, and you know how I loathe that word, "but we're having some trouble waking him up from the anaesthetic."

I'm sure my own heart stopped beating. "What do you mean?"

"We can't get him to breathe on his own. His heart rate is very slow. He's still on a respirator. Has he ever had trouble with anaesthetic before?"

"He's never had surgery before! I don't know! Is it serious?" I could feel panic rising in my chest. I wanted to run to his bedside and shake him awake and tell him to quit being an ass and wake up! I jumped up off my chair—almost forgetting that I only had one leg and couldn't run to the recovery room to be with my husband. Just then, a nurse came out and told us that Rick was finally awake. I let myself exhale, and realized I'd been holding my breath as I started to cry tears of relief.

Dr. So excused himself and said he had other patients to monitor but would check on Rick later. The nurse led me to Rick's side. He looked groggily at me and gave me his sweet, lop-sided grin, "Hi, honey. Did you miss me?" I kissed him softly and was amazed at all the wires and lines hooked up to my husband and shocked at the blood-filled urine bag attached to the bed.

Later on, I asked Rick what he could remember about the surgery after we had kissed goodbye in the waiting room. He said he filled out some more forms and was led to a bed then introduced to one of Dr. So's surgical team who drew some lines on his abdomen. Rick laughed and said it was to make sure the surgeon knew where to cut. He was wheeled into the operating room where Dr. So greeted him warmly and introduced him to the surgical team. The next thing Rick remembers was the anaesthesiologist placing the mask over his face and counting backwards, 100, 99, 98 ... and waking up in the recovery room completely unaware of the drama unfolding in the waiting room or the worry he had caused his care team.

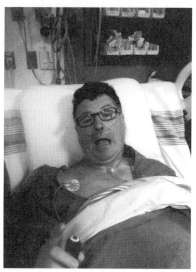

They kept him in recovery overnight with round-the-clock nurses to make sure his heart didn't slow down again. Surprisingly, he said there was very little pain, but he still enjoyed the next two days with the morphine drip very much.

Rick is actually clowning around with the morphine activator in this photo. He reported little pain from the surgery.

Chapter Five

Recovery—Ask and Ask Again

Rick spent one day longer in the hospital than many prostatectomy patients because of the difficulty he had waking up from the anaesthetic. His surgery was on Tuesday, May 1, and he was discharged on Friday, May 4.

There is one thing that happened at the hospital that I think needs to be shared. Rick isn't circumcised. That's not unusual in itself but it is if the staff didn't make a note of it on his chart. The day after his surgery, I watched as the nurses cleaned his surgery site and catheter and noticed that his penis looked weird—not because there was a catheter hose coming out of the end of it, but because the foreskin was pulled back. I asked the nurse, "Um, is his penis supposed to look like that?"

I guess I should have been more specific because she answered, "Yes, it's just swollen from the surgery and catheter." I didn't think it looked too swollen. It just looked oddly discoloured, as if a thin grey rubber band had been slipped under the penis head and was causing it to turn purple, but I figured I was no expert.

The next day, I watched again as the nurses cleaned and tended to Rick's private area. By now, my normally shy husband no longer turned red with embarrassment. As a matter of fact, Rick's modesty no longer existed. He was resigned to exposing his privates to any nurses or doctors who needed to take a look. Although the morphine was keeping him pain-free, his penis looked awfully sore to me. I noticed that the grey band was decidedly bigger than it had been the day before and the purple hue was deeper. This time, I decided to ask the nurse if she realized that Rick was not circumcised. She looked surprised and checked his chart. Nope. No mention of him not being circumcised. She looked a little alarmed and said she'd make sure to ask a doctor to come and take a look.

We spent that third day walking up and down the halls. No doctor came to look at his penis while I was there. They took him off the morphine and we were both surprised and pleased that he wasn't having more pain. Rick was also getting the hang of manoeuvring in and out of bed with his urine bag. It was approaching day four after his surgery. He was scheduled to be discharged in the morning but the head of his penis was now *very* swollen—and the grey ring was looking more like the size of a small glazed doughnut. The ring looked weepy and the head of the penis was so swollen and purple it looked almost black. After too many sleepless nights, I was exhausted and needed to get back to my hotel bed but, in case the doctors arrived to see him before I arrived back at the hospital in the morning, I had left Rick a list of questions that I wanted answered before bringing him home. At the top of that list was:

Check penis—foreskin has been pulled back since surgery—is it okay?

This question was followed by a short list of other concerns I had, such as when to change the dressing; when he could shower;

when would the catheter be removed; what could and couldn't he do around the house; and was vacuuming out of the question for a while?

Sure enough, a team of doctors arrived to go over his discharge and offer some home-care suggestions before I finished checking out of the hotel the next morning. Dr. Mike Robinson, the anaesthetist, led the team. Rick picked up my list and said, "My wife has some questions to go over with you." As he read out my first question, Dr. Mike lifted the sheet and had a look at the problem. So did the team. Unexpectedly, Dr. Mike grabbed Rick's penis in his big fist and squeezed hard. Rick almost fainted as lightning bolts of pain shot through from his groin all the way to the top of his head. Dr. Mike didn't miss a beat.

"So, what other questions does your wife have on that list for me? Go ahead. Read the list." And he continued to squeeze, harder.

"Holy crap! I can't focus my eyes, let alone read!" Rick exclaimed as he broke into a sweat. The care team's eyes all widened at the scene unfolding on the bed in front of them. Rick thought he might pass out because the pain was so intense. And still Dr. Mike's grip on his manhood didn't lessen but whatever he was hoping to happen obviously wasn't happening fast enough.

"Get me some KY, would you?" Dr. Mike calmly asked one of the interns. When the lubricating gel arrived, he temporarily relinquished his vice-grip on Rick's swollen member, and applied a generous dollop of KY to it. Rick initially thought the worst was over, but no such luck. With another determined squeeze, Dr. Mike compressed the foreskin and Rick swears he could almost hear an audible "pop" when the foreskin slipped back over the head of his penis where it belonged. The fireworks going off inside

Rick's head as this task was being performed rivaled those of any Fourth of July or Canada Day Celebration, I'm sure, but the flood of relief when Dr. Mike let go was beyond words.

"There you go! The big guy's got his hat back where it belongs." Dr. Mike seemed very pleased with himself. How could such a small piece of skin cause so much trouble and pain?

We are laughing now—well, actually, I was laughing when Rick told me about it later that morning when I came in—but it wasn't funny to Rick at the time. I think I laughed so hard that I actually peed my pants (a feat that gets a lot easier the older I get by the way!).

Rick was very animated when he described the action I had missed. He grew sombre though when he told me how serious things could have been if he had been discharged without rectifying the situation. Lack of circulation to *any* part of the body causes big problems.

Rick squeezed my hand and was only half kidding when he said I had saved his life again.

All joking aside, if you are *not* circumcised, be sure to mention this fact to your medical team before your surgery and be sure that the foreskin is returned to its normal, upright position after the catheter has been inserted.

Chapter Six

Recovery—
Home at Last

The trip home was uneventful. Rick left the hospital with his catheter attached and handled the highway bumps surprisingly well. He loved the fact that he could drink a large coffee and didn't need to stop enroute for a pit stop, "Hmm, a guy could get used to one of these things!" He was only half-joking, I think. I was just thankful that he didn't seem to be in a lot of pain and still had his sense of humour after the morning's foreskin torture.

When we got to Chilliwack he wanted to stop at the EI (Employment Insurance) office to file for medical leave but he was in his pyjama pants and was toting a rapidly filling bag of blood-tinged urine attached to a long hose coming out of his PJ pant leg. He was not quite dressed appropriately to make a public appearance, so I parked the car in front of the large EI plate glass windows and ran in.

Rick needed to sign some forms in person, but, bless the government rules, even though they could see him waving from the car just steps away from their desks, they insisted that he had to come *in* and sign the papers. They wouldn't let me take them to him. I wrestled with the notion of bringing him in his jammies but thought perhaps he'd suffered enough indignation for one day. We

rescheduled for the fol-
lowing week.

Rick settled into the
home routine nicely. His
comfy blue housecoat
became his wardrobe
of choice. He seriously
loved that catheter. He
thought it was just won-
derful to be able to sleep
through the night with-
out having to get up to
pee. He also loved that
he could have two cups
of coffee in the morning

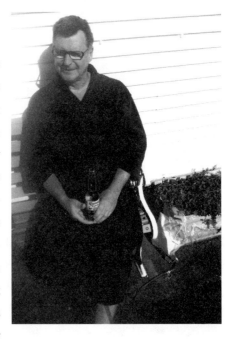

and a few beers at night and never have to leave the couch for a pee
break. But, sadly, all good things apparently must come to an end.
Poor Rick.

Ten days after his surgery we went to see our family doctor,
who removed Rick's staples and catheter. She took the staples out
without any incident. Rick is a fast healer and Dr. So had done a
beautiful job. Then came the catheter. He had been dreading the
procedure so he was very happy when it came out without any
trouble but—surprise, surprise—he promptly peed the moment
the tube was removed. Our lovely Doctor Julia passed him a pad
and explained, "Not to worry. That often happens until the bladder gets used to working again." Whew. We breathed a collective,
but short-lived, sigh of relief because we soon discovered that
many prostatectomy patients never regain full bladder control. It

takes patience, practice, and perseverance. We weren't prepared for this part. Not at all. We made a pit stop on the way home from the doctor's office—but this time it was to the drug store to stock up on Depend® underwear and other adult continence aids. Rick was mortified so I went in alone while he waited forlornly in the car wondering how the hell his life had come to this.

After frustrating days of constant dribbling and having no sensation that he even needed to urinate, Rick was fit to be tied. So that's what we did. We went online and discovered this marvellous invention for stopping the flow of urine. A penile clamp! We didn't hesitate—we ordered it and had it rushed to us. When it arrived we found that it was essentially a $200 device that clamped below the head of the penis to close the ureter tube so it wouldn't dribble. It was kind of like putting a kink in a garden hose. Remember doing that when you were a kid and remember what happened when you released the kink? Stand back folks—looks like we could be in for a shower! It was ridiculous and seemed slightly dangerous. But the theory was sound—if you pinch off the leak the pee won't dribble. The clamp does work but it also makes the bladder *very* lazy and we found out that it would only serve to make the problem worse if used on a regular basis.

I would only suggest one of these devices if corrective surgery would kill you and Kegel exercises won't work. Rick decided he would rather wear incontinence pads or protective underwear than a giant clothespin clamped on his penis. So much of Rick's recovery would prove to be trial and error. And there were more than a few trials ahead.

I belong to the Rotary Club of Chilliwack and had a Rotary function to attend on Saturday, May 12. Normally we would have attended the event together, but Rick did not want to go out so soon after his surgery, so I went alone. As he held the front door open for me, he wrapped me in his arms and gave me a long, sweet kiss goodbye. He brushed my ear with his lips and seductively whispered, "Hey honey, you know what?" I waited for him to say that he thought I looked beautiful, or that he wished he could go with me, but instead he let out a long, slow sigh and softly whispered, "I'm peeing my pants right now."

"Well, that's romantic!" I started to giggle and before long we were both laughing until the tears ran down *both* our legs! He has been blessed with the most wonderful sense of humour and that gift has carried us through the worst of trials.

Unfortunately, Rick is not a very good patient and he didn't enjoy feeling like an invalid. While I was at my event, he thought that perhaps a little exercise would be good for him rather than just sitting around on the couch waiting to be well again. For all who are reading this, remember you need time to heal so don't rush the process. Once again, we were about to learn this tidbit of wisdom the hard way.

Rick decided to go for a long, leisurely walk. It felt good to get out in the fresh air and he was very proud of himself but he certainly paid for it the next day when he complained that his testicles felt like they were the size of basketballs! They weren't that big but they were so sore he couldn't walk, sit, lie down, or even move without pain. He had a paralyzing pain in his left thigh. We wondered what on earth could cause these excruciating symptoms so we phoned Dr. So looking for answers. We were worried that something had gone dreadfully wrong.

Dr. So explained it simply, "When the prostate is removed the ureter tube is stretched when it is reconnected. When you stand for long periods, the weight of the testicles pull on that incision causing pain and swelling." The solution? Wear tightie-whities, not boxer shorts, and don't stand for extended periods! Tight underwear lifts and supports the testicles so that their weight doesn't aggravate the surgery site. The pain running through his thigh wasn't such an easy fix.

Apparently, some men experience nerve damage after the surgery which manifests almost like sciatic pain, but not where sciatica normally appears. Rick's nerve pain runs along the centre of his thigh emanating from his left testicle. His left testicle, even one year after the surgery, often feels swollen to Rick, even though it is not. It's just incredibly tender to touch and the nerve pain in his thigh seems to come and go at random—but in retrospect, it usually occurs after overexertion or wearing boxers for a few days in a row. Seems Rick has had a hard time replacing all his boxers with sensible undies, and still pays the price with pain.

Rick was certainly experiencing his share of trials along with his errors, but thank goodness for Prostate Support Groups. They are a wealth of information. We went to a meeting on June 7, and were given the name of a nurse at the Abbotsford Hospital who ran a continence clinic. She had already worked with almost every man at the meeting and they all blessed her for her help. Her name is Nelly Kaye but everyone calls her Nurse Nelly. We made an appointment to see her on June 20. It was a very long two weeks waiting to see if she could offer some solutions. *(She provided us with the information in the Need-to-Know section on how to do Kegel exercises properly.)*

We had a dinner date booked with our oldest son and his wife.

It was a lovely, warm day and Rick opted to wear an incontinence pad rather than the full protective underwear. We were learning so much about recovery after prostate surgery and what we learned that day is that an incontinence pad won't hold two beers without some spillage. When you can't feel that you have to pee and you hate to go to the bathroom when you're having fun, you are just setting yourself up for trouble. I looked at Rick as he stood up and we both realized that his jeans shorts were soaked. We cut our visit with the kids short. Rick was crestfallen. It was beyond mortifying to pee your pants in front of your children. His visit with Nurse Nelly couldn't come soon enough.

On Father's Day, I was the keynote speaker at our local Prostate Awareness/Father's Day Walk/Run event. Rick was determined to do the walk with his two boys by his side. He did the five kilometers that day wearing his Depend undergarment and even the rain didn't dampen his spirits. He walked proudly as a survivor, flanked by his two tall, handsome sons. A renewed determination filled him that day. He would do all he could to get better and the first thing to do was to see about getting his unruly bladder back under control.

I think Rick will always remember his first meeting with Nurse Nelly because what he didn't realize when we made the appointment was that she was a very attractive former acquaintance from high school! Prepare for another humbling experience.

"Hi. I'm Nurse Nelly. What can I help you with today?" She was warm, welcoming, and wonderful. We exchanged pleasantries and small talk before getting to the reason behind our visit. At some point in the conversation it dawned on Rick that he remembered her from his high school days. He looked at me and his eyes widened as he slowly realized that he was about to get naked in front of not just another medical professional but a woman he actually knew! I understood just how much of his modesty he had lost over the past weeks because he sucked in his stomach, pulled his shoulders back, and hardly blushed as he bared himself.

In no time at all, she had Rick hooked up to a machine that measured the strength of his Kegel and spent some time teaching him what a proper Kegel exercise feels like. It was no wonder he hadn't had any success with them. He had been doing them wrong the past few weeks. You know you're desperate for help when you're okay with having a beautiful woman you went to school with see you stark naked, allow her to hook electrodes to your most special places, and are thrilled to receive her accolades when you can stand up without peeing on the floor. Bless you, Nurse Nelly.

Rick was now on the road to regaining his dignity along with his bladder control but the next hurdle would prove to be a lot harder to jump over. Would we ever be able to make love again?

Chapter Seven

Recovery—Back in the Saddle Again

Dr. So hit the nail on the head when we first sat down in his office and he opened the conversation with, "Well, I bet you're wondering about erections." As a matter of fact, next to surviving the actual cancer diagnosis, it was one of our primary concerns.

I pray a lot. I pray for all sorts of things actually, but I was nervous and skeptical about putting my wish for Rick to achieve an erection into a prayer. Does God care what we do in the privacy of our bedrooms? I believe that He does, or He wouldn't have made it so much fun. So, with a little trepidation, I added a prayer every night that Rick's nerve-sparing surgery would, in time (*sooner* rather than later, please God), have him back to his former self.

As mentioned earlier, Rick and I enjoyed an active sex life and that was one of our favourite ways to show our love for each other. If you've read the book, *The Five Love Languages,* by Gary Chapman, you'll know that people have different ways of expressing love. There are basically five ways to express love, according to Chapman, and these are: through the giving and/or receiving of gifts, quality time, words of affirmation, acts of service, and physical touch. Rick and I both speak the same languages in that the first method we both respond to is acts of service, followed by physical touch, words of affirmation, quality time, and, last on both our lists, is gifts. This probably explains why we've stayed married since 1982 while many of our friends' marriages have crumbled. If you don't speak the same language or know which language your spouse responds best to, it makes it much harder to stay in love and happily married.

At our 30th anniversary party, our oldest son summed it up beautifully when he said, "I've seen more acts of spontaneous affection than I ever wanted to from my mom and dad..."

It's not that we can't keep our hands off each other, it's just that we both enjoy a good back scratch, a caress on the arm, back rub, head scratch, kiss, or a hug whenever we can. We will often touch each other as we pass by in the kitchen or hallway. It's our way of saying I LOVE YOU without actually saying I LOVE YOU. It works for us because physical touch is a love language we both speak. It might not be yours, so this part of our story might not interest you. Feel free to skip it if it makes you uncomfortable.

When Dr. So told us that Rick was a good candidate for the nerve-sparing surgery, we were very happy. We had read that if a person enjoyed an active sex life before the surgery, they were even more likely to be able to recover the ability to have an erection afterwards. It sounded easy because Rick was enthusiastic and optimistic that he would return to normal quickly after the procedure; but that darned prostate gland has a mind of its own. It may be small but it's mighty important to a man's sexuality.

We knew that sex was out of the question as long as the catheter was in place, but Dr. So suggested we start stimulating the penis as soon as we could after the catheter was removed. Did you know a man can have an orgasm without having an erection? We didn't! It was a pleasant surprise for both of us (well, probably more pleasant for Rick than it was for me).

In *Things You Need To Know And Helpful Tips,* I've included a link to get detailed instructions for gentle stretching and massage of the penis from a wonderful resource pamphlet about penile rehabilitation after pelvic cancer surgery or radiation for men from www.sexualityresources.com—reprinted with their permission.

At first, I dutifully massaged Rick's penis every day after the catheter was removed, but I found it very frustrating. For more than thirty years I'd been rewarded with an instant response that showed me how much he welcomed my touch. Now that the visual response of a rising erection was removed I found that the foreplay was unrewarding for both of us. It seemed to me that when they removed his prostate they also removed his desire to have sex. He seemed to have forgotten that I didn't have *my* emotional drive removed, and I felt unloved and neglected while he was recuperating. As Reanne Booker has pointed out:

> Very little is known about the partner's experience (not much research has been done in this area). Partners often feel neglected, unloved, unattractive, etc. As health care professionals, we definitely need to do a better job of supporting partners.

As Dr. So had suggested, I waited about six weeks before attempting to give Rick a manually stimulated orgasm. We had a follow-up appointment in mid-July and I really wanted to see if Rick was able to climax, so we could have some good news to share with our wonderful surgeon. To our surprise, Rick did have an orgasm.

There was no ejaculate though, and he experienced an odd, but not entirely unpleasant, burning sensation in the perineum area at the point of climax. It was entirely different than the orgasms we were both used to and I found that reaching an orgasm took much longer for him. Quickies were out of the question.

On July 12 we returned for a follow up visit with Dr. So. He was glad to hear that Rick was able to have an orgasm, and I was very glad when he said that it wasn't entirely up to me to take charge of Rick's penile rehabilitation. He told Rick that it was important for him to massage his penis daily, in order to stimulate the flow of oxygenated blood needed to keep the nerves and blood vessels healthy enough to achieve an erection. For me, that meant that intimacy could become a pleasure and not a chore! For Rick, that simply meant spending a little more focused time in the shower.

After a prostatectomy, because the tube that is the ureter is cut above and below the prostate gland before being stretched back together and reconnected when the gland is removed, a man's penis loses up to one-quarter of an inch (or one centimetre) in length. Rick says that's not true at all—he swears he lost at least an inch. I will say it's a shock to see someone who woke up every morning with his compass proudly pointing the way to the toilet now wake up with his needle pointing forlornly at the floor instead.

Sex was important to us before the surgery, but I think you must realize that things can change drastically for some men after the procedure. Rick says it almost felt like he'd been castrated. Watching love scenes on TV did nothing for him; seeing scantily clad women on the beach wouldn't even make him turn his head; kissing and touching seemed to almost annoy him. I found it incredibly lonely, and I missed the intimacy we had in and out of our bedroom more than I ever thought possible. What on earth was I going to do? I did a lot of praying, I can tell you that. Finally, we sat down and talked.

Rick is an intelligent, sensitive, handsome, and loving man. He was going through a very difficult transition himself, and it was incredibly hard for him to care about what someone else was coping with, when he had so much on his plate already. But a marriage is a partnership, and if one partner isn't happy it can ruin the relationship. Sitting down and discussing real feelings and fears is difficult no matter how long you've been married, but we did, and it was the turning point that made all the difference.

Rick was so focused on his own healing that he couldn't see how lonely I was without his physical touch. After our talk, he started stroking my arms again, scratching my back, kissing just for kissing's sake, and not with the expectation of sex to follow! In essence he brought the intimacy back into our relationship, even without the sex. The best news is that sex eventually has followed the intimacy.

Many men don't understand that women don't necessarily want just sex and that we actually enjoy the cuddling, kissing, and caressing part equally and, in some cases, more. However, sex is still important and there are ways to bring that act back into the bedroom, when the spirit is willing, and you're up for a bit of an adventure.

After our follow up with Dr. So, Rick and I went on a five-week *Choosing to Smile* book signing and speaking tour in July, 2012. In Calgary, we had lunch with Reanne Booker, the wonderful nurse practitioner we'd met at the cancer conference in Saskatoon before Rick's surgery. She suggested an external penile pump could really help with stimulating the blood supply to the penis and facilitate his rehabilitation. We knew nothing about this sort of device but Reanne assured us that they could be effective.

The following week, we were at the West Edmonton Mall doing a *Choosing to Smile* book signing and, as luck would have it, there was an Adults Only store just around the corner. We walked to it after my event, and Rick, being far too shy, opted to sit on a bench and eat ice-cream while I boldly stepped into another world and giggled to myself as I remembered an old joke Rick had told me years earlier, made even funnier because of the way he told it:

> Have you heard about the little old lady who went to a sex shop and asked the clerk in a quivering voice, "Excuse me, do you have any of those vibrating things that are, ohhhh, about this long and about this wide?" The clerk assured her they carried them, and with relief the little old lady said, "Oh good! Then maybe you can ssshhhhooow me how to shhhuuut it off!"

Apparently, people of all ages use sex toys, but they certainly aren't for everyone.

Don't be shocked. Don't be nervous. Don't be surprised. I repeated to myself before entering. And yet, here I was standing inside a whole other world feeling shocked, nervous, and more than a little surprised! WOW! It shouldn't come as any big surprise that people have all sorts of kinks and twists, but it is a little shocking and nerve-wracking when you've always considered yourself pretty straight. I decided that nobody knew me in Edmonton, so I could feel free to ask the clerk for exactly what I needed.

The woman seemed surprisingly normal and was very helpful. I bought an inexpensive penile pump, lubricating jelly, and a penis ring that was supposed to hold the blood inside the erect penis. The total came to a little more than $100, and the kind clerk said it would work.

When we got home I was eager to try the pump and see if it would do what it was supposed to do. It didn't. I guess you get what you pay for. Reanne had mentioned that a medical grade pump would cost upwards of $500 but with Rick not working yet we were reluctant to spend that kind of money on something non-essential.

In theory, the vacuum system of the pump draws blood into the non-erect penis and creates an erection. The pump we bought didn't create an airtight seal so it worked a little but not enough to create an erection stiff enough for penetration. Still, it did increase the blood flow, which is what was needed, and allowed Rick to do his therapy on his own, outside of the shower. I had had grander visions, I suppose. Still, Reanne had ignited a bit of hope in Rick again and encouraged us to try other means of intimacy in the bedroom.

You don't need to go to an adult store to buy "bedroom toys" as there are other options for sexual intimacy. I'm not going to tell you what Rick and I do in the bedroom but the point is, my husband was willing to step outside his comfort zone to make sure that my needs were met if he wasn't able to meet them. Intimacy in the bedroom *is* important and means different things to different people.

One of the things that helps a lot is knowing a few tricks ahead of time. For example, don't expect the fire to light, if you don't have any spark to begin with. Before you even think about going to your bedroom, you can start setting the mood simply by holding hands, touching each other in gentle, non-sexual ways, kissing each other hello and goodbye or for no reason in particular, giving compliments, encouragement, and letting your partner know that, even if he can't rise to the occasion, his touch is still welcomed. Bedroom toys aren't for everyone. When Rick discovered that he could satisfy my needs even without having an erection, it was a very happy day in our household!

Rick says he's not sure what magic is in that little walnut-sized prostate gland but it can very effectively emasculate and humble a man when it is removed. He used to say that he could walk through the grocery store, look at a couple of cantaloupes, and get an erection. All that changed after his prostatectomy. He hardly noticed my breasts anymore, it seemed. But, after his surgery, he found that he could get emotional watching sappy commercials. He felt more in touch with his feminine side than he had ever wanted to be!

Studies show that the sex drive can come back if the nerves are spared. It just takes patience, time, effort, and perseverance. Some of the literature we've read says it can take up to four years after surgery to regain erectile function. Sometimes we both just wanted to give up and say, "to heck with this!" but then his penis would involuntarily flicker and renew our determination to continue rehabilitation exercises. It was frustrating for me not to be able to arouse my husband in the way that I'd grown used to over the past three decades, but it was even more frustrating for Rick. We had to find ways to connect outside the bedroom.

I gained back fifteen pounds of the eighty-five pounds I had lost the year prior to Rick's surgery because we went out for frequent lunch and dinner dates to make up for the quality time we used to spend behind closed doors. It was worth the weight gain just to be able to hold hands across a dinner table and re-kindle some romance. Many men and women don't realize that intimacy isn't just found in a bedroom.

Chapter Eight

What Works and What Doesn't

There are many toys/appliances on the market that are designed to help men with erectile dysfunction. Some work. Many don't. Sometimes simpler is better.

Penile massage is important to help regain erectile function. Many men find that if they get down on their hands and knees the blood flows into the penis much easier and makes the therapeutic massage more effective. At least it looks like it's working because there is significant growth in girth and length and that is encouraging for both partners. Some men, even after taking Viagra*, Cialis*, or health food store supplements, will not be able to become erect enough for penetration. But don't give up. There are other options like the injection of medication, or even a penile pump implant, if all else fails.

On October 4, 2012, Rick and I went for what we thought was our last option. We went to see a doctor at the Prostate Health Centre in Vancouver who would instruct us on how to use needle therapy to gain an erection. A friend of ours has great success with this method so we thought, for the sake of this book, we at least should give it a try (even though Rick is less than fond of needles!).

We sat in the office waiting for the doctor. Rick was pale and his blood pressure was through the roof. He wanted to be anywhere but in that small, cramped doctor's office. To top it off, the doctor showing us the procedure was a young and attractive woman. Poor Rick. More women have seen his private parts since his surgery than when he was single and looking for women to show his private parts to!

The doctor was very professional, but I had to laugh when she had a look at Rick's penis and made a comment about how he needed a haircut. It looked like a ball of wool had exploded in his nether regions—funny I'd never noticed that before. She drew a syringe with a dose of saline in it. We needed to use saline to practice and make sure we were comfortable with the procedure. We would save the real medicine for the privacy of our bedroom.

Rick looked at me and said, "Listen, the only way I will be able to do this is if you give me the injection. There's no way I can do it, Glenda." I had given our dog insulin injections for years so I was pretty sure I could handle poking his penis. Bless my wonderful husband for being a good sport.

The injection is made with a tiny needle into the side of the penis and contains medication that relaxes the smooth muscle of the penis to increase blood flow. It usually takes about five minutes from time of injection for erection to occur and it lasts from thirty minutes to two hours. If it didn't work we would have to return for a follow-up visit to ensure we were receiving a proper dosage of the medication.

The advantage to the injections is that they can produce completely normal erections and, aside from having a needle phobia, they are easy to prepare and administer. This treatment option does not involve surgery, is only minimally painful and can be used any time. Although self-injection therapy can cost up to $25 per injection, it is much less expensive than surgery. The disadvantage to injection therapy is that the reports of satisfaction with this technique range between 50 percent and 70 percent. Some men report that the injections cause urethral pain and burning. Injections should be limited to once or twice a week to minimize risks of scars or penile damage. The most serious complication of penile injections is priapism, a painful condition where the erection persists and does not go away. These are all things we needed to consider before trying injections. And if injections don't work, there are still other options.

I slid the saline filled needle into the side of Rick's penis under the watchful eyes of the doctor. Rick flinched. I giggled. Rick wasn't happy that I was having way too much fun at his expense. The doctor said I was a pro, but I didn't feel confident that I could do it at home with the real deal. It was important not to have any air in the syringe. It was important to inject the medicine into the right vein. It was important to remember to alternate sides. There were too many important details for either of us to feel comfortable doing this just for the sake of an erection. There had to be another option.

The doctor asked us if we had tried a penis pump. I told her about the sex shop purchase that was an abysmal failure but she assured us that a medical grade pump would be worth trying. She also mentioned again that Rick would need to manscape (shave off the pubic hair) or the pump wouldn't seal properly. She wrote out the prescription for the medication for the injections and also wrote out one for a penis pump which we could purchase in the pharmacy located in the Prostate Centre. The pump would cost us $500, but we did the math and figured out that, at $25 for one injection, we would only have to make love twenty times to have it pay for itself. We are apparently very practical people. We bought the pump.

We followed the instructions for using the pump very carefully. Rick was determined that this had to work. (Personally, I think he was terrified I'd make him do the needle therapy if it didn't.) Is it oversharing to tell you that, on Saturday, October 19, we had liftoff? Yes folks, we did indeed have a happy ending! No needles. No surgical implants. No pills. No potions. Just a medical-grade penis pump. God answers all sorts of prayers in all sorts of ways, you know!

Chapter Nine

Life Goes On

A friend of ours had a radical prostatectomy in his early fifties and had a penile pump surgically implanted. His wife candidly told me that sex has never been better for them because now he can last until she's had enough and, because there is no ejaculate, there is no mess to clean up. On the other hand, another friend of ours in his mid-fifties had the non-nerve-sparing surgery. He has absolutely no desire for any type of sexual interaction and yet his wife and he had enjoyed a very active pre-surgery sex life. They have come to terms with the effects of his surgery and she, like many other women, is content to take care of her own sexual needs herself. I am not that gracious.

I like intimacy. I like cuddling and kissing. You don't need a penis for these things. Many men think that the only reason to cuddle or kiss their spouse is to culminate the act with intercourse. Sometimes cuddling and kissing can lead to that but, and this is going to come as a surprise to some men, it's not always what women want. Sometimes, we just want to be held and caressed gently as we fall asleep in the arms of someone we trust and feel safe with. A penis is important but it's not the centre of the universe—it's merely a nice perk that comes with most men's pre-prostatectomy package.

On Father's Day, 2013, Rick walked in the Prostate Awareness event again flanked by our two sons. This time, he wasn't wearing any protective undergarments and shaved about thirty minutes off

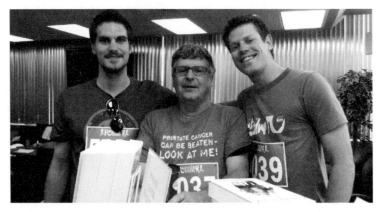

his last year's time—in other words, they weren't dead last! What a difference a year makes.

Rick and I have certainly had our ups and downs (no pun intended). Like most married couples, some days we would gladly trade each other in for newer models but most days we are at peace with each other, content, and comfortable together. Some people think that life has given us more than our share of challenges but we wouldn't trade our troubles for anyone else's. Prostate cancer isn't an automatic death sentence and it certainly isn't the death of intimacy in a relationship either. Rick's diagnosis gave us an opportunity to grow and learn together and even more than that, it provided even more incentive to live life to the fullest and not let any opportunity to express love pass us by.

We hope that, by sharing our story, you feel braver, more informed, and capable of coping with whatever adversity comes your way. We found that if we remembered to count our blessings, to communicate our wants and needs, to be patient with each other and if we always remembered to love, then we would survive and handle the trials together. Prostate cancer is not the end. It's simply a detour.

Epilogue

Rick and I are looking forward to a busy time ahead, speaking and travelling to spread the word about prostate health and awareness. Because I am obviously physically disabled, people know I've likely experienced some medical challenges in my life but Rick's surgery is invisible, and people have no idea that his life has drastically changed because of his cancer experience. We want the stigma of speaking about prostate cancer to be removed. We don't want any other couples to have to search for a book that explains what a diagnosis of prostate cancer means. We want doctors to hand their patients our book and say, "Oh, and here's a book you might want to read. It will answer your questions honestly and give you a sense of direction."

When the pathology report came back after the prostatectomy, Rick's Gleason Score had jumped to a grade 8 and 9 from the original biopsy result of a 6 and 7. His cancer was incredibly aggressive and Dr. So said we were very fortunate to have made the choice to have the surgery when we did. The pathology report indicated that there was no sign that the cancer had spread beyond the prostate. We know that we are very fortunate to have caught Rick's prostate cancer early. We also know that, even though making love isn't the same as it once was, we are still very lucky to have regained a semblance of what we thought was lost forever.

When I speak at conferences and to groups people often ask me what we would do differently. I've compiled a little list:

- Learn to do the Kegel exercises properly and practice them religiously before the surgery.
- See a continence nurse or specialist as soon as possible.
- Tell the surgeon, nurses, care team, everyone, if you are *not* circumcised.
- Wear tight underwear that supports the testicles after the surgery—no exceptions.
- Don't go for long walks or engage in strenuous exercise. Let the internal incision of the urethra heal thoroughly. Follow your doctor's recommendations.
- Take small doses of Viagra˚ or Cialis˚ following the surgery if they spared the nerves—no matter what the cost.
- Buy a *good* medical grade penis pump and use it as soon as the catheter is removed or as soon as your surgeon says it's safe to do so.
- Communicate honestly with your spouse about what you're feeling and what the personal expectations, wants and needs are for both of you.
- Be extraordinarily patient with each other.

To send your feedback, or to book Glenda as a speaker, contact her at info@glendastandeven.com and visit her websites:

> www.iamchoosingtosmile.com
> www.glendastandeven.com
> Mailing Address:
>> 9872 Candow Street
>> Chilliwack, BC
>> V2P 4K4
>> Canada

Things You Need To Know
and
Helpful Tips

Much of the following information is taken from the online resource:

Information for Men Newly Diagnosed with Prostate Cancer

Urologists at the Vancouver Prostate Centre

Martin E. Gleave, M.D., FRCSC, FACS

Director of the Vancouver Prostate Centre

S. Larry Goldenberg, OBC, M.D., FRCSC, FACS

Alan So, M.D., FRCSC

Peter Black, M.D., FRCSC, FACS

Patient Education Services

B. Joyce Davison, Ph.D., R.N.

Address

Gordon & Leslie Diamond Health Care Center

Level 6, 2775 Laurel Street

Vancouver, BC V5Z 1M9

Canada

Phone: 604-875-5006; Fax: 604-875-5024

www.prostatecentre.com

What Is a Prostate Gland?

Basic Anatomy of the Prostate

The prostate is one of the male sex glands. The other major sex glands in men are the testicles and the seminal vesicles. Together, these glands store and secrete the fluids that make up semen.

The prostate, about the size of a walnut, lies just below the bladder and surrounds the upper part of the urethra. The urethra is the tube that carries urine from the bladder and semen from the sex glands out through the penis. As one of the sex glands, the prostate is affected by male sex hormones. These hormones stimulate the activity of the prostate and the replacement of prostate cells as they wear out. The chief male hormone is testosterone, which is produced almost entirely by the testicles or testes.

What Are the Warning Signs of Prostate Problems?

Please note that the following symptoms could indicate that you may be experiencing Benign Prostate Hyperplasia (BPH) which is a condition that affects the prostate gland. "Benign" means that it is not cancer and "Hyperplasia" means enlarged. When the prostate becomes enlarged over time due to exposure to male hormones it can press down on the urethra and act much like a clamp on a garden hose. This can block the flow of urine and make it difficult for the bladder to empty. BPH is not the same as prostate cancer but it does manifest many of the same symptoms.

Enlarged Prostate Symptom Checklist

Check off all the statements that apply to you.

- ☐ Urination has become more difficult than it used to be.
- ☐ Many times I feel I have to push to start the flow of urine.
- ☐ I awake two or more times at night to urinate.
- ☐ When urinating, the stream stops and starts again several times.
- ☐ After I urinate, my bladder does not feel fully empty.
- ☐ When I feel the need to urinate, it is harder to wait than it used to be.
- ☐ My urinary stream is weaker and less forceful than before.
- ☐ My symptoms are having a negative impact on my daily life.

If you checked off even one of the above statements, you could have an enlarged prostate. Take the list with you to your next doctor's appointment to discuss the symptoms.

For more information, visit www.MyBPH.ca

Many of the early warning signs of prostate cancer are identical to the signs of having an enlarged prostate gland. That is why it is so important to get checked as soon as you notice any change in your urination pattern.

What Is the Gleason Scale?

According to the Canadian Cancer Society website www.cancer.ca

Gleason classification for prostate cancer

The most common grading system for prostate cancer is the Gleason classification system. It is used to describe how aggressive a prostate cancer tumour is, and how likely it is to spread. The Gleason classification is used only for adenocarcinoma, the most common type of prostate cancer.

The Gleason classification reflects how different the structure of the tumour tissue is from the normal prostate gland structure. It was based on a grading scale from 1 to 5 (but 1 and 2 are no longer used). The scale is used to describe the patterns of the prostate cancer gland structure and growth as they appear under a microscope.

Grade 3

A grade of 3 means the cancer cells still form well-defined glands but they are invading the surrounding prostate tissue.

Grade 3 tumours are well differentiated.

Grade 3 is considered favourable. It indicates less aggressive cancer.

Grade 4 – intermediate between grade 3 and 5

Grade 5

The cancer cells no longer form organized glands and instead resemble a random organization of very abnormal cells.

Grade 5 tumours are poorly differentiated.

Grade 5 is considered less favourable. It indicates a more aggressive cancer.

To assign a Gleason score (also called a Gleason sum), the pathologist looks at the biopsy sample of the tumour to find the two most common types of glandular growth patterns within the tumour. A grade from the scale is given to each of these two patterns. The two grades are added together to get the total Gleason score. For example, if the grade given to the most common growth pattern is 3 and the grade given to the second most common growth pattern is 4, the total Gleason score is 7.

The Gleason score is always between 6 and 10. Higher Gleason scores indicate more aggressive tumours. Most prostate cancer tumours are low and intermediate grades (Gleason score 6–7). Gleason scores below 6 are not usually given because it is difficult for the pathologist to determine with certainty that the lowest grade tumours are in fact cancer.

Read more: http://www.cancer.ca/en/cancer-information/cancer-type/prostate/pathology-and-staging/grading/gleason-classification/?region=on#ixzz2m11iGNjh

---

*Note from Glenda: It is important to *know* your Gleason score and understand what it means after your biopsy. It is equally important to know your PSA numbers after your annual blood work and understand what those numbers mean. Don't be afraid to ask!

How to Do a Kegel Exercise Correctly

according to The Source—Your Guide to Better Bladder Control information pamphlet

Pelvic floor muscle Kegel exercises

Developed by Dr. Arnold Kegel, these exercises are designed to strengthen the muscles of the pelvic floor so that the bladder is kept in place and the urethra stays shut tight. Kegel exercises work best for people who have stress or mixed incontinence, but anyone can try them, even as a preventive measure to keep your pelvic floor muscles strong.

How to do them

- Stand, sit, or lie down with your knees slightly apart. Relax.
- Find your pelvic muscle. Imagine that you are trying to hold back urine or a bowel movement. Squeeze the muscles you would use to do that. DO NOT tighten your stomach or buttocks.
- *Women:* to make sure you've got the right muscle, insert your finger into your vagina while you do the exercise. You should feel a tightening around your finger.
- *Men:* when you tighten the pelvic floor muscle, your penis will twitch and contract towards your body.
- Tighten the muscles for 5 to 10 seconds. Make sure you keep breathing normally.
- Now relax the muscles for about 10 seconds.
- Repeat 12—20 times, three to five times a day.

Stick to it! You should begin to see results after a few weeks. Like any other muscle in your body, your pelvic muscles will only stay strong as long as you exercise them regularly.

If you're having a hard time doing Kegel exercises, your healthcare professional can teach you how to do them correctly. He/she may even suggest a tool or device to help make sure you're using the right muscles.

Your doctor may also suggest biofeedback, a training technique that's used to monitor the contraction of the pelvic floor muscles as you do your Kegel exercises. Biofeedback uses a machine that records the contractions of your muscles and translates the movement into a visual signal that you can watch on a monitor. Some people find this helpful in learning how to do Kegel exercises correctly.

Biofeedback training is usually given in a hospital or private clinic by a physiotherapist, doctor, nurse or trained technician, but you can also buy or rent a machine to use at home.

What You Need to Know About Penile Rehabilitation

The following segment is used with permission from the Woman's Touch Wellness Series www.sexualityresources.com

Introduction

Health problems like diabetes, heart disease, and cancer may have a direct impact on a man's ability to achieve a penile erection. Many men can take important steps toward improving, maintaining, or recovering erectile function, as long as they understand how the penis works, and which techniques improve function. This article outlines techniques that can improve your specific situation.

How Do Erections Happen?

Sexual arousal is a response to stimulation produced by several mind and body systems working together. An erection is one sign of a man's sexual arousal, when the clitoral body swells with blood and the penis becomes stiff and hard. (Women get erections, too, but since their clitoris is placed differently in their genitals, you see the vulva swell instead.)

Erections require

Intact physical structures: The clitoral body inside the penis is a unique structure. There is a fiber-like flexible shell on the outside that stretches during erection, small curled blood vessels that occasionally open to let oxygenated blood in, and stretchy sacs that hold blood during erections. It is the stretch, tension, and blood flow that makes a penis hard and erect. All of these parts have to be healthy, flexible, and free from inflammation or scarring in order to create a firm erection.

Specific biochemistry

Small curled blood vessels in the clitoral body relax in response to a chemical called nitric oxide, which allows blood to flow into the penis. Nitric oxide can be produced either by stimulation of nerves of the pelvic plexus, or in the walls of the clitoral blood vessels when they are stretched and massaged.

Low overall body inflammation: Nitric oxide is a sensitive chemical, and doesn't work when we eat junk food. Really. It also doesn't work if we don't get daily exercise. Eating a healthy diet and walking every day supports sexual arousal, helping nitric oxide do its work.

In a healthy person, these different systems work together to create a penile erection. The loss of function of any part of the system means that attempts at sexual arousal—and erection—may be unsuccessful.

Finally, it's important to get complete deep sleep every night. During the dreaming phase of sleep, nerves activate swelling of the penis approximately 4-6 times per night. Penile swelling exchanges oxygenated blood for non-oxygenated blood within the clitoral caverns, and is critical to maintaining the health of the clitoral body. The final swelling of the penis each night results in the "morning erection" that many men wake up with—this is a good indication that all physical systems and structures are functioning properly.

Why Do Erections Stop Happening?

Erectile dysfunction (ED) is the inability to develop or maintain a penile erection sufficient for sexual penetration. It's fairly common, occurring in 21-46% of all men. Common causes include metabolic dysfunction or surgical trauma.

Metabolic disorders—Heart and blood vessel disease, metabolic syndrome, and diabetes are the most common causes of ED. The inability to get reliable erections is an early sign that something isn't working right, and is often a man's first warning that he is at risk for a heart attack within 3–5 years.

Surgical Trauma—Another common cause of ED is anything that damages, stretches or cuts the pelvic plexus nerves deep in the pelvis, which commonly happens during surgical or radiation intervention for prostate, colon, or rectal cancer. Prostate cancer therapies cause ED (radiation therapy 43%; radical prostatectomy 58%), because the therapies damage nerves, blood vessels, and/or clitoral components. Minimally-invasive surgical approaches may reduce complications right after surgery, but they still increase post-surgical ED.

Some Men Have Both—It's common for men with prostate cancer to have pre-surgical metabolic ED. Men who had trouble getting erections before the surgery often have more difficulty recovering after the surgery, because the underlying erectile dysfunction impairs recovery from surgery.

Erectile Dysfunction from Metabolic Disorders

All portions of a man's erectile system are sensitive to metabolic disorders due to an inflammatory Western lifestyle. Eating a diet high in refined carbohydrates and low in healthy oils and proteins, plus limited voluntary exercise is a very dangerous combination for sexual health. Sexual health requires the peak performance of cardiorespiratory fitness, and many men aren't aware of the effects of their daily choices.

Penile Rehabilitation is a group of specific techniques that can help maintain men's sexual health. However, men with metabolic dysfunction need to go one step further. If your health status continues to include poor blood sugar control, high carbohydrate food choices, and a lack of routine exercise, etc., you may not be able to benefit from the Penile Rehabilitation program to its fullest. A widely known treatment, the group of medications like Viagra*, may not be available to you because your health prevents their use.

Make a careful assessment of your priorities:

- Does your sexual health matter enough for you to make significant food changes?
- Does a half-hour of walking every day still seem like a burden when it may mean the difference between reliable erections or not?
- Your erections are accurate indicators of your overall health.

If they aren't working regularly any longer, your health is already less than you deserve. You can use techniques #2, 3, and 4 in this article. But in addition, we suggest you make serious changes towards better health.

Injury after Prostate Cancer Surgery

The path of the pelvic plexus—the delicate nerves that carry sexual arousal information between the penis and the lower spine—curves around the prostate, colon, rectum and bladder. When surgery is performed on the prostate, some nerves will be cut and some will be stretched. Even the most skilled and careful surgeon cannot avoid stretching the nerves. Stretched nerves become stunned, and although they are complete and in place, they cannot function until they recover. Though some men's nerves may recover soon after surgery, the recovery process may take up to three years for others.

In the meantime, when the nerves stop working, oxygen-rich blood will stop flowing to the clitoral body inside the penis, and scarring can occur. It's important to keep blood flowing to the nerves, small blood vessels, and the clitoral body inside the penis, so that the oxygen exchange still happens. This will allow the structures to work when nerve function recovers.

We can't know when nerve recovery will occur, so it's worth it to facilitate blood flow to the penis for the whole three years after surgery. Fortunately, the techniques we outline here will help improve oxygen-rich blood flow to the penis even when nerves can't do the work.

First Experience After Surgery

Surgery has a negative, time-limited effect on men's erections that all men need to be aware of. A man goes into surgery with the penis length and function he is used to. When he wakes up after surgery, he will see the urinary catheter that has been placed inside his penis, which helps drain urine and keep the passage from the bladder to the penis open. This catheter also artificially stretches the length of his penis.

The clitoral bodies inside the penis won't get any oxygen-filled blood after the surgery. Unavoidable nerve stretching and lack of oxygen will cause the penis to shrink, and when the catheter is pulled out (often right before hospital discharge), the penis may appear to be only half of its previous length. Shocking as that is, a man with good underlying function may recover his regular morning and on-demand sexual erections within days or weeks.

Sometimes, more extensive stretching and nerve shock or damage occurs, which happens during many pelvic surgeries. In this case, waiting alone will not get erectile function back. Working to restore erectile function becomes an important part of a man's post-surgical recovery.

Goals of Penile Rehabilitation

Penile Rehabilitation (PR) is the process of regaining erectile function, erectile length and girth, and hardness. The main goals of PR are to:

- Increase daily oxygen exchange to the penis, and
- Maintain length and girth of the penis such that full erection size and hardness are possible once the nerves have recovered.

As mentioned earlier, consistent daily blood flow bathes the erectile nerves and blood vessels with oxygenated blood, keeping tissue healthy and preventing scarring of the clitoral body inside the penis. If appropriate, medications should begin immediately after returning home from surgery. Try to begin the physical components of PR as soon as you feel physically comfortable enough to touch your penis, or within 2 months after surgery, whichever is sooner. There may be discomfort as internal scars heal; if any part of the process is uncomfortable at first, wait a few days before starting or restarting your program. However, if there is pain with PR, stop and consult your health care provider.

Remember: the sooner a man begins PR, the more likely the success. Men who had surgery within the last three years will still benefit from PR, particularly if they occasionally have soft morning erections. PR will help on-demand therapies work better. PR can also create erections hard enough for sexual penetration even when the nerves have been permanently damaged by using Vacuum Erection Devices with a erection/cock ring.

Techniques of Penile Rehabilitation

There are seven possible therapies used to help men regain erectile function after prostate cancer surgery. Since clinical studies show that combining different healing techniques increases the chance of success, we recommend using the following four techniques together:

    #1: A low nightly dose of PDE-5 Inhibitor medication

    #2: Gentle stretching and massage of the penis

    #3: Use of a Vacuum Erection Device (VED) twice daily

    #4: Pelvic Floor Muscle Exercises

Three additional techniques require the supervision of a medically-trained urologist: a) prosthetic implants, b) MUSE-medicated urethral system for erections, and c) Intercavernosal injections (ICI) into the clitoral caverns of the penis. Because of the possible risks and side-effects, they are not described here, but you may discuss them with your health care provider.

Technique #1: Use a nightly dose of PDE-5 Inhibitor medications
Phosphodiesterase-5 Inhibitor (PDE-5 I) medications like sildenafil (Viagra˚) are not only useful for on-demand sexual activity.
Small nightly doses are significantly more likely to help deliver
oxygenated blood to the inside of the penis while you dream, and
to move your recovery forward. These medications help your natural nitric oxide biochemistry work to facilitate erections, particularly while you sleep. Some men notice that nightly low dose use
helps them recover spontaneous functional erections.

The preferred daily medications are:

- Sildenafil (brand name: Viagra˚) begin at 25 mg per day at
  bedtime, or
- Vardenafil (brand name: Levitra˚) begin at 5 mg per day at
  bedtime.

You should slowly work your way up to the maximum rec-
ommended dose for either medication (sildenafil up to 75mg; or
vardenafil up to 10mg; at bedtime), but always start at the lowest
dose to reduce any side effects you may experience. If the side effects of the higher dose become uncomfortable, resume the original low dose. Ask your health provider about any serious side
effects. Since most health insurance plans do not cover daily doses
of PDE-5 Inhibitors, ask your health care provider to write your
prescription in the highest available dose, and split the pills to cover daily dosing.

PDE-5 I medication will not guarantee preservation of girth
and length. Scarring may occur before erections begin to happen regularly on their own. Only Vacuum Erection Devices will
preserve girth and length, so they should be used in combination
with PDE-5 I medications.

These medications should be taken right before bed on an empty stomach to encourage natural penile swelling during sleep. If you wake up with soft morning erections, this is a sign that the rehabilitation is working. This may not happen right after surgery, but is a good sign if it does.

Common Side Effects of PDE-5 Inhibitor Medications include:
Diarrhea; dizziness; flushing; headache; heartburn; stuffy nose; upset stomach. Discontinue use and seek medical attention right away if any of these SEVERE side effects occur when using PDE-5 Inhibitor medications: Allergic reactions (rash; hives; itching; difficulty breathing; tightness in the chest; swelling of the mouth, face, lips, or tongue); chest pain; fainting; fast or irregular heartbeat; memory loss; numbness of an arm or leg; one-sided weakness; painful or prolonged erection; ringing in the ears; seizure; severe or persistent dizziness; severe or persistent vision changes; sudden decrease or loss of hearing; sudden decrease or loss of vision in one or both eyes.

Technique #2: Gentle stretching and massage of the penis
Stretch activates the vessels that bring blood into the penis, and massage decreases the risk that your penis will become unused to, or uncomfortable with, sexual touch. Achieving erection is not the goal, but a soft erection at the base of the penis is a positive sign.

The massage should be pleasurable, not painful. Using the following steps, your massage should take about 10 minutes per day:

Select a personal lubricant (for more information, please look at our article on Personal Lubricants). A lubricant should make massage more comfortable, and offer a balance between slide and friction.

- Holding the tip of the penis with one hand, use your other hand to gently squeeze and massage the shaft toward the body (removing blood from the penis).
- Then, gently stroke and stretch the penis away from the body (allowing blood to flow back in). Some urologists recommend gently squeezing all parts of the penis up and down the length of the shaft, from all directions.

Note: Do not sharply bend the penis—this could cause injury.

This massage should be gentle and comfortable. If you can, consciously focus on any massage motions that feel good, without making a hard erection your goal. Most men's penises will remain soft during the massage, so remember that recovery takes time.

Technique #3: Vacuum Erection Device (VED)

Vacuum erection device (VED) therapy has a very high rate of consumer satisfaction (92%), and most importantly, is the only therapy that preserves both the length and the girth of the clitoral body inside of the penis. The pump's vacuum stretches tissue inside the clitoral body, while breathing/pumping blood in—and out—of the penis. The goal is to gently draw oxygenated blood into the penis, then allow it to flow out again.

Stretching the penis as far as it will go, or holding a maximal stretch for too long, can reverse the benefits of vacuum pumping—new blood stops flowing in with sustained high pressure. Men who have metabolic ED respond well to vacuum therapy alone, but may have even better responses if they can also take a daily dose of PDE-5 I medication 1 hour before using their VED.

Depending on the fit of the VED, a testicle may be drawn up into the vacuum chamber; using a pump with a soft adaptive sleeve at the end of the vacuum tube will help prevent this, while making for a more comfortable fit.

Remember, when using a VED for Penile Rehabilitation, you are not trying to create an erection (if this is your goal, see Intimacy & Pleasure, below). Vacuum pressure stretches the clitoral body inside the penis so that it doesn't "forget" how elastic it needs to be with full erections. VED therapy is the only way to provide this internal stretch.

We describe two restorative pumping methods here. Before pumping, perform the self-massage and gentle stretching of the penis as described above. Both pumping methods draw fresh (oxygenated arterial), and stale (desaturated venous) blood into the penis, so the color of the penis will be bluer than a spontaneous erection. This is ok, since the new blood:

a) adds more oxygen than was there before,

b) exchanges inflammatory fluids in the pre-pumped blood, and

c) stretches the clitoral tunic sheath and maintains its flexibility.

It is normal to see your penis turn a slight blue color, but don't hold the blood in too long. When the pump vacuum is released, follow with the self-massage technique to coax the blood back out.

Restorative pumping methods include *Double Pumping*, and *Pump-3-Release*. Double Pumping is easier to do—just be sure not to pump too quickly. The Pump-3-Release Method takes some counting, but this variation more effectively moves blood in and out of the penis.

Double Pumping:

1. Lubricate penis and gently perform a self-massage.
2. Insert penis into chamber, then adjust chamber against the body to create a vacuum seal.
3. Slowly and gently pump to create a comfortable vacuum. This should take about 5 minutes.
4. At maximal comfortable vacuum level, pause for 10 seconds, then release the pressure.
5. Remove penis from pump, then holding the tip of the penis, massage from tip to base, gently squeezing blood out of the penis.
6. Repeat steps 2–5.
7. Repeat morning and night, or 3 times per day as time allows.

Pump-3-Release:

1. Lubricate penis and gently perform a self-massage.
2. Insert penis into chamber, then adjust chamber against the body to create a vacuum seal.
3. Slowly pump 3 times. Release the vacuum and count to 5 (one-banana, two-banana, three-banana, etc…).
4. Slowly pump 3 times. Again, release the vacuum and count to 5.
5. This time, slowly pump up until you reach the maximal comfortable vacuum level without pain.
6. At your current maximum level, HOLD and count to 5.
7. Fully release vacuum, then take a deep breath.
8. Remove the penis, then hold the tip and massage from tip to base, gently squeezing blood out of the penis.
9. Repeat morning and night, or 3 times per day as time allows.

Technique #4: Pelvic floor muscle exercise

The pelvic floor is a sling of muscles that surround and anchor the base of the penis, helping to hold blood in the penis during erections. Exercising these muscles will strengthen them, allowing you maintain firmer erections. These muscles pulse with orgasm, so orgasms will be easier to feel when they are strong and flexible. Pelvic Floor therapists developed exercises specifically to help men restore function of their pelvic floor muscles. Try to do these exercises as often and as consistently as possible. It's fine to miss a day or a session—just get back to the routine when you can.

To locate the correct muscles, stand and look down at the penis.

See if you can make the base of your penis move down and in. Sometimes it helps to feel the muscles by placing your hand against your perineum (the area between your scrotum and your anus), or by pretending to stop the flow of urine. If the penis moves up and down, then you are contracting the correct muscles.

Your health care provider or a physical therapist can help you locate the muscles if you have trouble on your own. To begin these exercises, find a comfortable reclining position, then:

1. Contract the muscles as firmly as you can and hold for a count of 5.
2. Release the contraction.
3. Take a deep belly breath and completely relax the muscles.
4. Repeat the contract-hold-relax-breathe cycle 5 times each session.

Do your exercises 3 times in the morning, and 3 times in the evening.

The relaxation portion of these exercises is as important as the contraction portion for two reasons. First, relaxation with a big deep breath allows blood to flow into the muscles, restoring oxygen and moving out any exercise-produced waste fluids. Second, muscle strengthening is most effective when the muscles are both strong and flexible, not tight and cramped. A deep belly breath allows you to completely relax the muscles.

Once your penis can visibly move when performing these exercises in a reclining position, try them while sitting, then standing, for three repetitions in each position in the morning and in the evening. You can also contract these muscles after urinating, to help strengthen the muscles that stop urine leakage. While walking, hold these muscles at half-strength for 10 steps, then relax for 10 steps, remembering to breathe during the session.

Intimacy & Pleasure

Many men who have had pelvic surgery or radiation are able to enjoy pleasure and orgasm without ever having an erection. This is important to remember, as men can enjoy many intimate activities without any erection at all. Some men choose to facilitate an erection by taking PDE-5 Inhibitor medication before sexual activity, and/or to use a Vacuum Erection Device (VED) and an erection ring to create an erection sufficient for penetration.

Full-dose PDE-5 Inhibitor

1. Sildenafil 25—75 mg. on an empty stomach 2 hours before activity, or
2. Vardenafil 5—10 mg. on an empty stomach 1 hour prior to activity.

Dosage: If you already take a PDE-5 Inhibitor daily and want to try for a full erection with only medication, you can take an additional dose of your regular medication. For example, if you take sildenafil 25 mg by mouth every night, you can take an additional dose of 75mg—bringing you up to the maximum dose of 100mg per day—2 hours before you are going to be intimate. (With vardenafil, you can take another 5mg dose 1 hour before sexual activity.) Remember to work up to a maximal dose. Higher doses may work better, but you will have more chance of headache, stomach upset, or other side effects. Talk with your health care provider for more specific information.

Communication: Full-dose medication requires a little planning and communication with your partner(s), since you need to take it before the heat of the moment. This doesn't have to be uncomfortable or awkward—try and find a way to talk with your partner about the medication, using it as a way to heighten the anticipation of sex. Letting your partner know in advance can help them feel included, and can lead to some fun foreplay ("I'll take my medication, we'll sit down to a candlelit dinner, and then move on to after-dinner delight...").

On-demand VED with Erection Ring

Vacuum erection devices (pumps) help create erections, even if a man does not have spontaneous nerve function. In other words, VEDs work even if your nerves will not bring blood into the penis by themselves, or if PDE-5 I medication isn't suitable for your health condition. You can use a VED with—or instead of—medication.

If you are using VED therapy to achieve an erection sufficient for sexual penetration, you'll need to place an erection ring at the base of the penis before you pump (see p. 17 for examples). When you have pumped the vacuum to your maximal comfortable penis size, tighten the ring to hold in the blood. The ring can be worn for up to 20 minutes, and it helps the erection stay firm by preventing blood from leaving the penis.

To use VED therapy for on-demand erections:

1. Warm a sexual lubricant that is compatible with the ring's material in a warm-water bath, or wrap the bottle in an electric heating pad.
2. Slip the erection ring over the opening of the pump's

chamber, or put an adjustable ring loosely around the base of the penis before inserting into the VED chamber.

3. Lubricate the penis, then gently stretch and massage.

4. Insert penis into chamber, and adjust chamber against body to create vacuum seal.

5. Pump either straight to maximum vacuum, or Pump 3-Count 5.

6. If you use an erection ring: when at maximal comfortable vacuum level, slip the ring from chamber to the base of the penis, releasing vacuum from chamber. This represents the beginning of the 20 minutes of ring use.

7. Proceed with intimacy, using warmed lubricant as needed.

8. Remove ring within 20 minutes, to allow new oxygenated blood to reach the clitoral body.

Note: After 20 minutes of use, the oxygen will be removed from the trapped blood in the penis, and without blood circulation some men notice that the penis becomes temporarily cold and discolored. If this is uncomfortable, you can warm your personal lubricant in a hot water bath, or remove the erection/cock ring and let blood re-circulate.

Don't use a erection/cock ring for longer than 20 minutes, since lower oxygen levels may scar the inside of the penis. This is worsened if a ring is used longer than 30 minutes.

In men who can ejaculate, an erection ring may impair ejaculation, cause pain during ejaculation or retrograde ejaculation. If this happens, choose an adjustable ring and loosen or remove it prior to ejaculation. Men who do not ejaculate (due to removal of the prostate) may find that a tighter ring is suitable, since it prevents involuntary urine loss during sexual activity.

Alternatives to Spontaneous Penile Erections

What if three years have passed since my surgery? What if I know that the nerves going to my penis are not going to work?

Sometimes the function of nerves that control erection of the penis are lost, either from a very extensive surgery, or a combination of other factors. If you do not have soft morning erections three years after the surgery, then you may no longer have spontaneous erections.

If you and/or your partner(s) decide that penetration is an important part of your intimacy, there are a variety of options. In addition to VEDs, erection rings, and medication, there are a variety of tools and accessories that men can use to help maintain a desirable level of sexual intimacy. These include special sleeves that fit over a non-erect penis, harnesses, and dildo combinations designed for men to wear, and vibrating toys.

Yes, it's an adjustment. Some men choose technology to meet their needs because the effort is worth it to them and their partners. Others feel it isn't worth the bother. It's a decision that only you can make.

For men who lose spontaneous erectile function after surgery, these tools can help you continue to create hard erections, and learn to pleasure yourself and/or your partner(s). If you work with these techniques for three years and are unable to regain spontaneous function, you also know that you've done what you can for your health, and can discuss further options with your health care provider.

For additional support and resources, men recovering from cancer can join their local **Man to Man Prostate Cancer** support group; contact the American Cancer Society by calling 1-800-227-2345 or visiting www.cancer.org, and locate a group near you.

Conclusion

Combining the techniques outlined here can help you rehabilitate your erectile function after pelvic surgery. Regular blood flow to the penis is important, even (and especially) when erections aren't happening like they used to. Many men lose spontaneous erectile capacity after pelvic surgery because they didn't know how to support their erectile function during the healing process. Although rehabilitation takes time and patience, many men do recover nerve and erectile function after pelvic surgery.

Pleasure for you and/or your partner(s) does not depend on your ability to create spontaneous erections. Intimacy is yours to define.